FULL BODY DETOX AND NATURAL CLEANSE BY TRADITIONAL METHOD

KSHAMA RAO

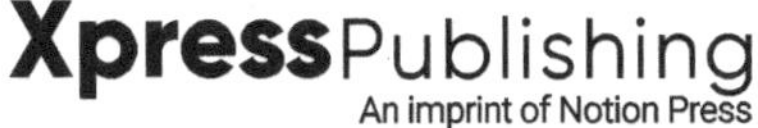

XpressPublishing
An imprint of Notion Press

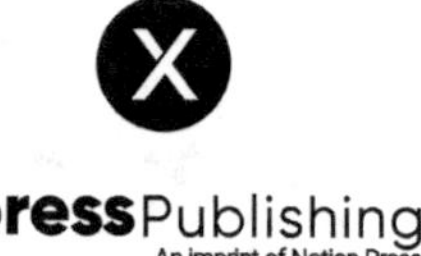

Old No. 38, New No. 6
McNichols Road, Chetpet
Chennai - 600 031

First Published by Notion Press 2019
Copyright © Kshama Rao 2019
All Rights Reserved.

ISBN 978-1-64760-593-3

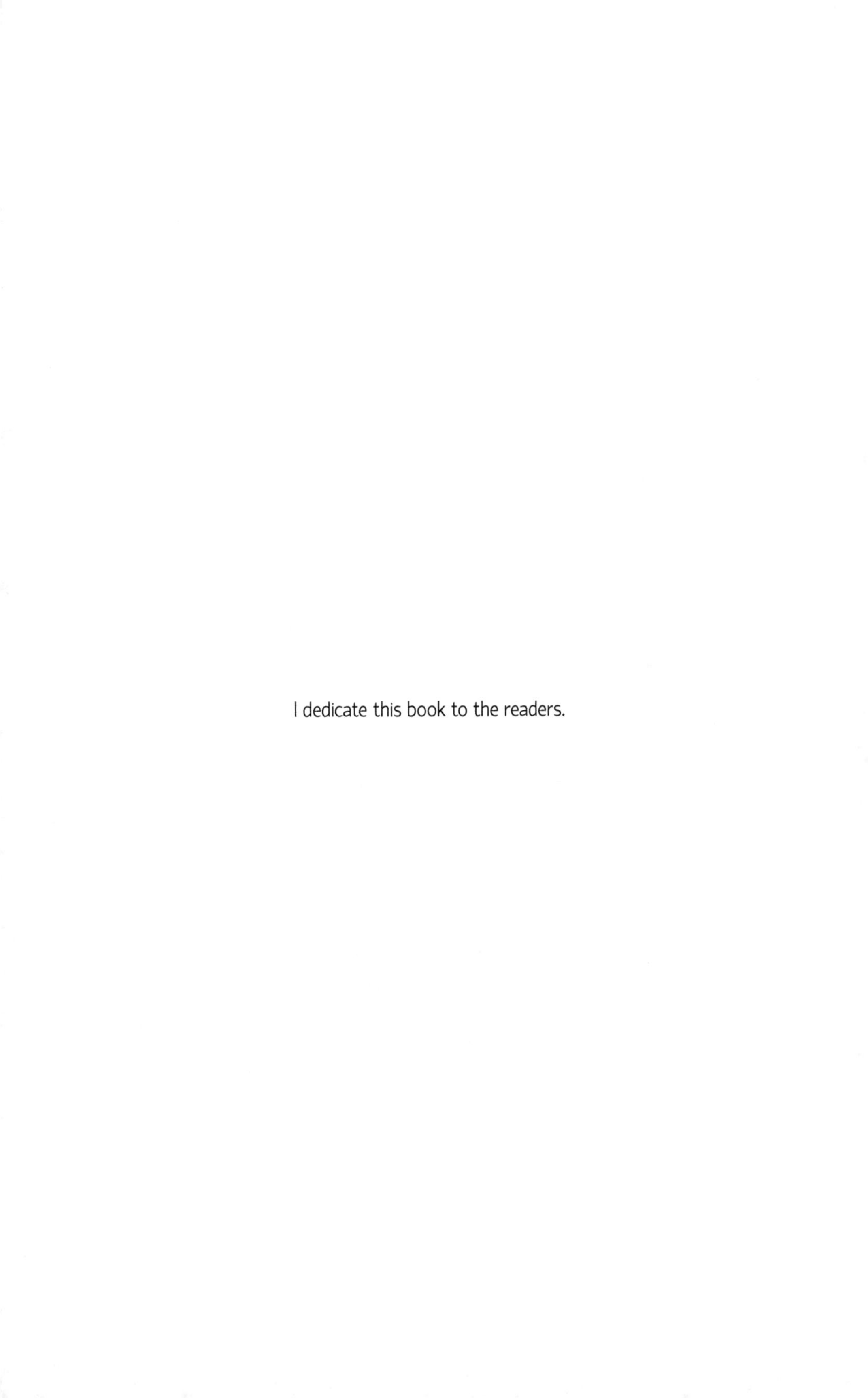

I dedicate this book to the readers.

Contents

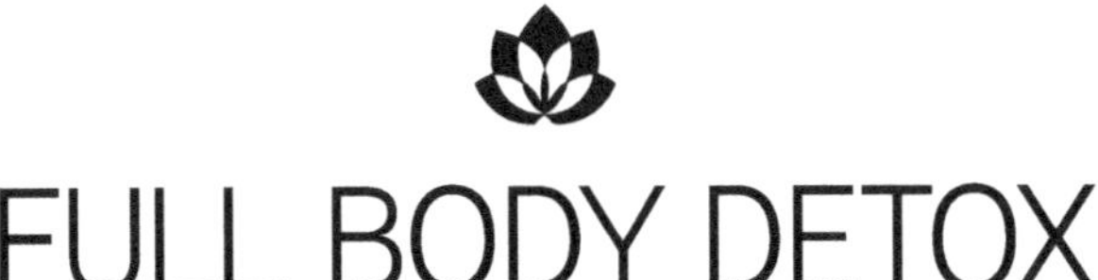

CHAPTER ONE

FULL BODY DETOX

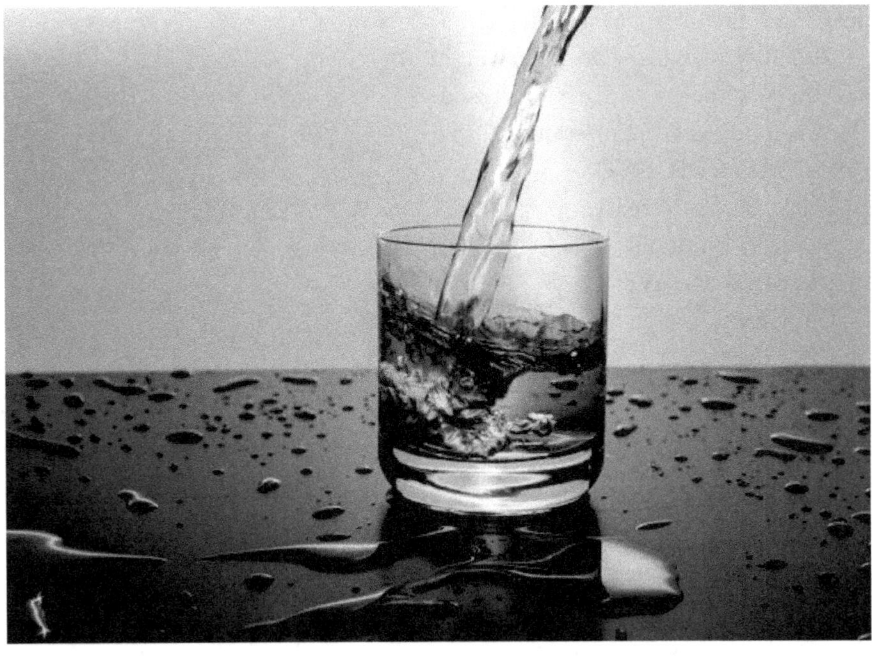

We live in a world, where toxins are everywhere. Pollutants, chemicals, heavy metals and processed foods affect our health negatively. Our body is working constantly to remove these toxins. The excess toxins are stored in our fat cells. Our vital organs come under pressure when we make unhealthy food choices, drink alcohol, consume too much caffeine or tablets and when we are under stress. Detoxification aids healing of your body.

SIGNS THAT YOUR BODY NEEDS DETOXIFICATION

You constantly feel stressed.

You experience headache or Nausea.

You experience bloating, cellulites or fatigue.

You are wheezing.

You have acne, puffiness in your eyes or dark circles.

You have urinary tract infections.

You have insomnia or mental fogginess.

Your digestion is troublesome.

You consume less healthy foods like processed foods, fried foods and sugary food.

You consume too much alcohol or caffeine.

You are exposed to harmful chemicals like carbon emissions, smoke, pesticides and artificial scents.

You are overweight or underweight.

You lack energy and are depressed.

Your body and breath stink.

BENEFITS OF DETOX

Prevention of diseases.

Stronger immunity.

Increased energy.

Glowing skin

Clear eyes

Mental clarity

Increased longevity.

Here are some natural ways to detox your body

SLEEP

Ensure that you get good quality sleep every night. Sleeping helps in the removal of toxins from your body and recharges your brain.

WATER

Water quenches your thirst and hydrates your body. It helps in regularizing the body temperature. Water transports waste products.

DIET

Reduce salt intake as it can cause bloating. Avoid processed foods. Eat probiotics like yogurt. Eat a diet rich in antioxidants like berries, vegetables and green tea. Reduce intake of sugar. Avoid alcohol and caffeine.

EXERCISE AND MEDITATION

Exercise helps you sweat. Sweating helps in releasing the toxins from your body. Meditation helps in relieving stress.

A COMPETE BODY DETOX

A complete body detox focuses on detoxing each organ. It removes harmful chemicals and toxins from your body. In this book, I have explained how to do a complete body detox by traditional method. A full body detox will help your liver and you will look young and graceful.

CHAPTER TWO

HOW TO DETOX YOUR BODY WITH AYURVEDA

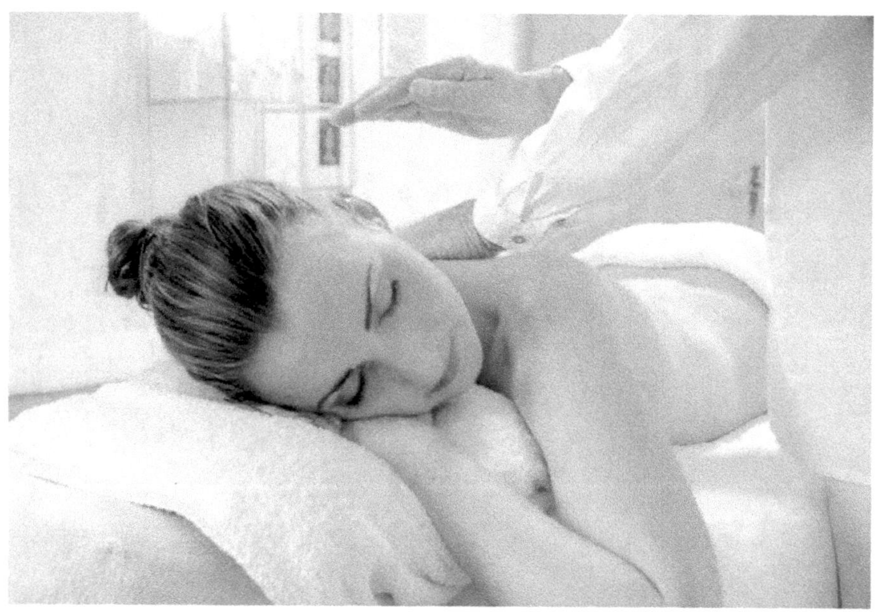

Unhealthy eating, having liquid and solid foods simultaneously, doshas (Vata, Pitta, and Kapha), weak immune system, Ama increases food, sedentary lifestyle, having irregular meals, poor digestion and insufficient sleep causes toxin formation in your body. Here are some tips to get your body detoxified.

PANCHAKARMA TREATMENT

Panchakarma treatment is useful to detoxify your body. Panchakarma treatment includes Ayurvedic oil massage, Kichari diet, steam bath, enema cleansing and other detoxification process. The process may last for 21 days.

DIET

Don't eat raw or frozen foods. Drink warm water instead of normal water. Avoid eating packed food, sugary food, colas and you should even avoid yogurt and honey. Consume Kitchari prepared from pulses, spices, rice, ghee and Moong dal. This is amazingly good for your gut health. Consume Triphala supplement.

ABHYANGA (WARMOIL MASSAGE) AND STEAM BATH

Full body oil massage is helpful in eliminating toxins. You can take a steam bath at your home itself. Be in the bathroom for a long while.

EXERCISE AND SLEEP

Feel nature by sitting in a park. Do yoga, meditation and walking in a park nearby. Sleep well for eight hours. It helps in detoxifying your body. Follow early to bed and early to rise technique.

CHAPTER THREE

HOW TO DETOX YOUR SKIN

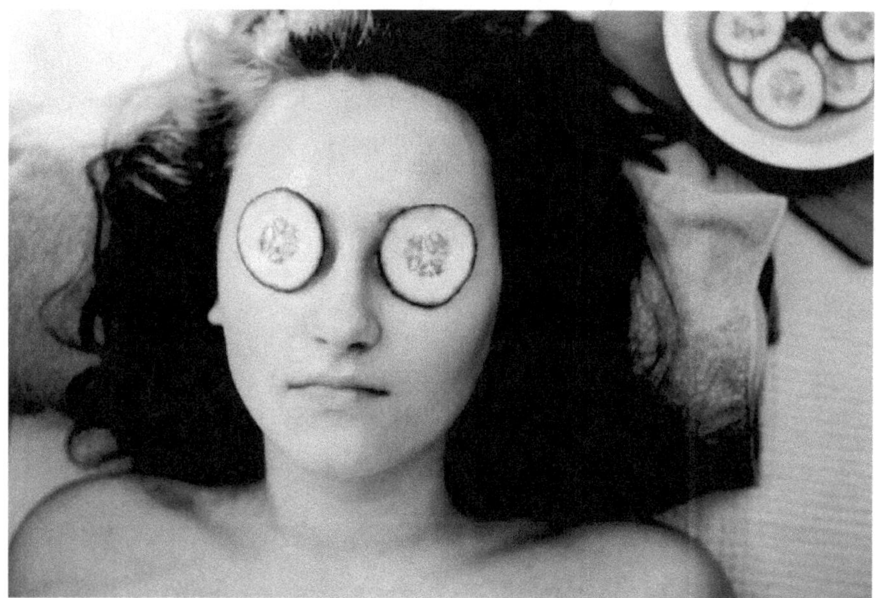

Some days our skin may look extra dull. It may be needing detox. Here is how to detox your facial skin.

CLEANSE

A skin detox requires cleansing in the morning and night. Use a cleanser suitable for your skin. It will clear all the build up.

SCRUB

You can use a coffee scrub to exfoliate your skin. Exfoliation helps in removing the dead cells.

FACIALS

Facials can clean out your pores and they are de-stressors. You can choose a facial pack suitable for your skin.

STEAM

Bring a pot of water to boil. Transfer this water to a wide bowl. Hover your face above the bowl. Drape a towel over your head to concentrate the steam on your face. Do this for ten minutes.

MUD MASK

Clay draws out impurities. Leave till it gets half dried. Don't wait to leave the mask till it cracks. It may strip off the essential oils from your skin. Apply the mask every alternate day to detox your skin.

HYDRATE YOUR SKIN

Serums should be used in the morning and at night. You can use sunscreen in the morning and revitalizing cream in the night. You should also apply a facial oil once in a week. If you have a sensitive skin you can apply Aloe Vera gel.

STAY HYDRATED

Drink lots of water. You should drink at least ten glasses of water in a day. This will keep your body hydrated and your skin moisturized. Water keeps your complexion glowing. It prevents wrinkles. Avoid tea, coffee, soda, sugary drinks and alcohol consumption.

DETOX THROUGH FOOD

Opt for alkaline rich fruits like watermelon, bananas and pears.

CHAPTER FOUR

MOUTH AND TEETH DETOX

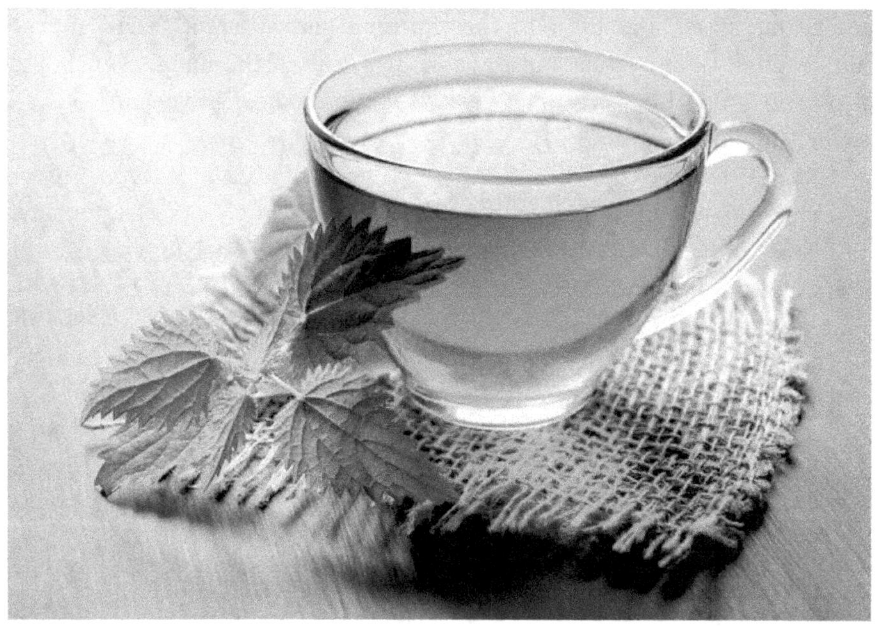

Mouth and teeth detox is as important to get rid of the toxins and chemicals. There are many daily routines that will help detox your mouth and teeth. Here is how to do the detox.

OIL PULLING

Oil pulling helps to say goodbye to toxins. It freshen ups your mouth. Coconut oil is best for oil pulling. You have to take a tablespoon of coconut oil and swish for ten to fifteen minutes. This will pull the toxins present in your mouth and whiten your teeth.

TONGUE SCRAPING

Tongue scraping is effective in removing bacteria and toxins from your mouth. You have to buy tongue scrapers and start scraping your tongue with it on a weekly basis. Tongue scrapers are easily available online for a reasonable price.

NON TOXIC TOOTHPASTE

Choose a chemical free toothpaste. Look for toothpastes that contain Eucalyptus, Neem and Peppermint.

CILANTRO

Drinking vegetable juice and cilantro juice is beneficial in removing the mercury and chemicals from our body. You should drink cilantro juice after your visit to the dentist as the fillings contain mercury and you might have been exposed to harmful X-rays while dental check up.

DRINK GREEN TEA

Green tea helps in improving brain function. It is useful in burning fat. It lowers the risk for diabetes and cancer. The catechin present in green tea is beneficial for gum and teeth health.

CHAPTER FIVE

HOW TO CLEAN AND DETOX YOUR LUNGS

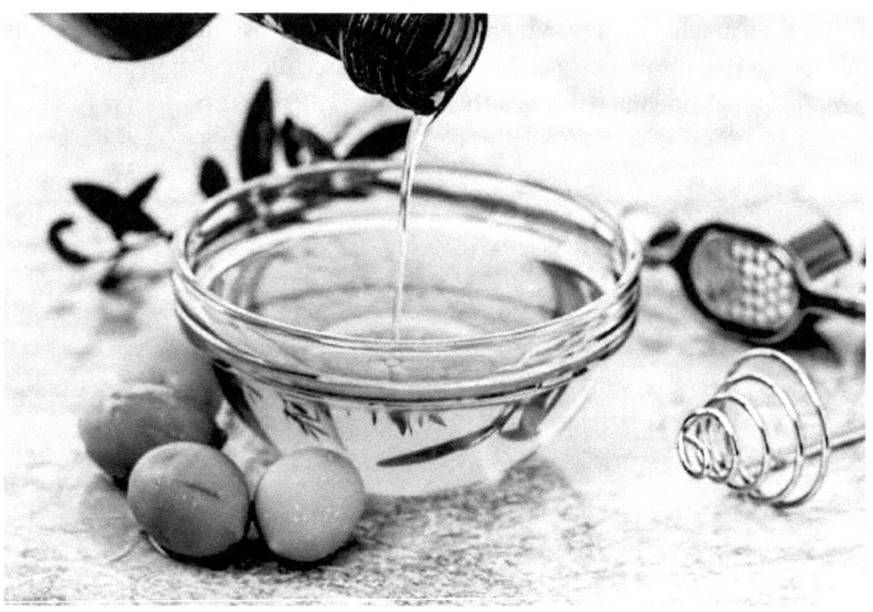

The main task of the lungs is to take oxygen and leave carbon dioxide. It is important to keep our lungs healthy.

A lung cleanse helps detoxify. It helps to cleanse the respiratory linings of the bronchial passage of lungs. It helps clear mucus in the lungs. Here are some methods to cleanse our lungs.

DEEP BREATHING

Deep breathing nourishes your lungs. It is helpful in reducing stress. Close your eyes and deep breathe five times. Hold your breath for a few seconds and exhale slowly. Repeat five to ten times. Do this breathing exercise twice a day.

CASTOR OIL

Castor oil helps in eliminating toxins from your lungs, uterus and liver. It reduces inflammation.

OREGANO

Oregano is rich in carvacrol and terpenes which act as a lung cleanser. It reduces inflammation. You can use oregano in cooking.

GINGER

Ginger can also detoxify your lungs and improve blood circulation. You can drink ginger tea twice a day.

PEPPERMINT

Peppermint can relax muscles of your respiratory tract.

IMPROVE AIR QUALITY

Chemical based air fresheners contaminate the indoor air. The carbon monoxide, formaldehyde and ammonia present in them can cause harm to your lungs.

LUNG CLEANSING DIET

Start your day by drinking a glass of warm lemon water. Eat foods rich in vitamin C like strawberries, tomatoes and oranges. Include antioxidant rich foods like garlic, turmeric and green tea. Avoid drinking coffee and alcohol. Avoid dairy products.

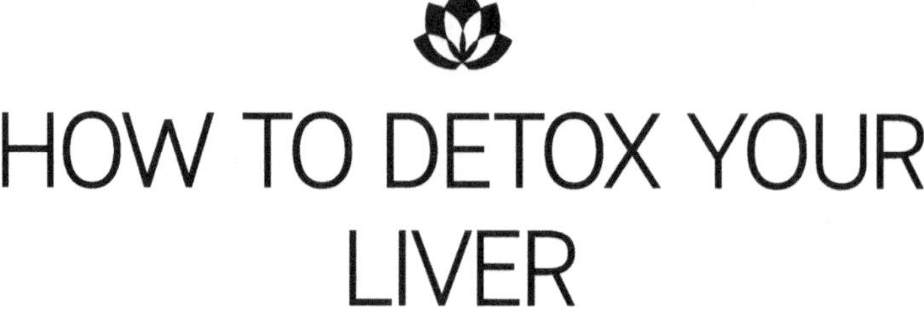

CHAPTER SIX

HOW TO DETOX YOUR LIVER

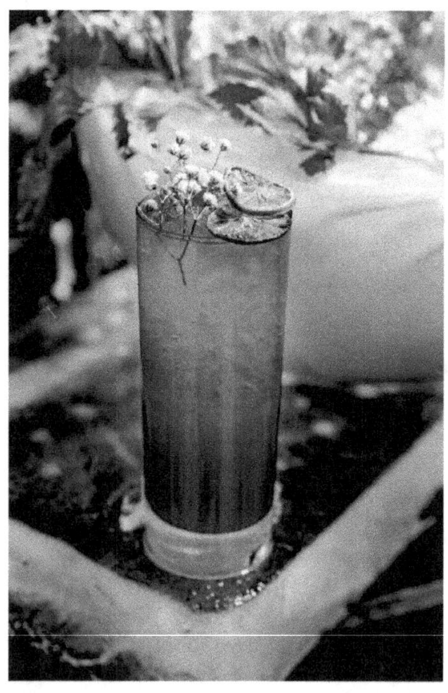

The liver is responsible for breaking down substances. It is your body's filtration system. It cleanses your blood. Here is how to detox your liver naturally.

INTERMITTENT FASTING

Intermittent fasting helps in reducing body fat and regenerates stem cells and your liver.

INCREASE YOUR INTAKE OF B VITAMINS

B Vitamins help in producing energy. B Vitamins can make your cells break down nutrients, more efficiently. This prevents fat accumulation around the liver.

INCREASE YOUR INTAKE OF VITAMIN C

Vitamin C is a powerful antioxidant. It can help fight inflammation. Vitamin C can help protect your liver from toxins and free radicals. It is easily broken down in the body.

BEETS

Beets contain betalains, which reduces inflammation and repair liver cells. They also contain, betaine, which helps liver cells to eliminate toxins.

MILK THISTLE

Milk thistle has antioxidant and anti-inflammatory properties. It stimulates the regeneration of liver cells.

DANDELION TEA

Dandelion is known for its cleansing properties. It also stimulates bile production.

CONSUME POTASSIUM RICH FOOD

Potassium intake is important for maintaining a healthy cardiovascular system, lowering bad cholesterol and blood pressure. Bananas and sweet potatoes are rich in potassium.

WATER

Water contains natural minerals. You can add lemon to your water to make it more alkalizing. Flushing your liver is like giving your body a pre wash.

EAT HEALTHY FATS

Your liver is responsible for producing bile that cuts down fats. Eat healthy fats like almond, walnut, hemp, flax, Chia, pumpkin seed, sunflower seeds and olive oil. Avoid vegetable fats and animal fats.

CHAPTER SEVEN

HOW TO DETOX THE PANCREAS NATURALLY

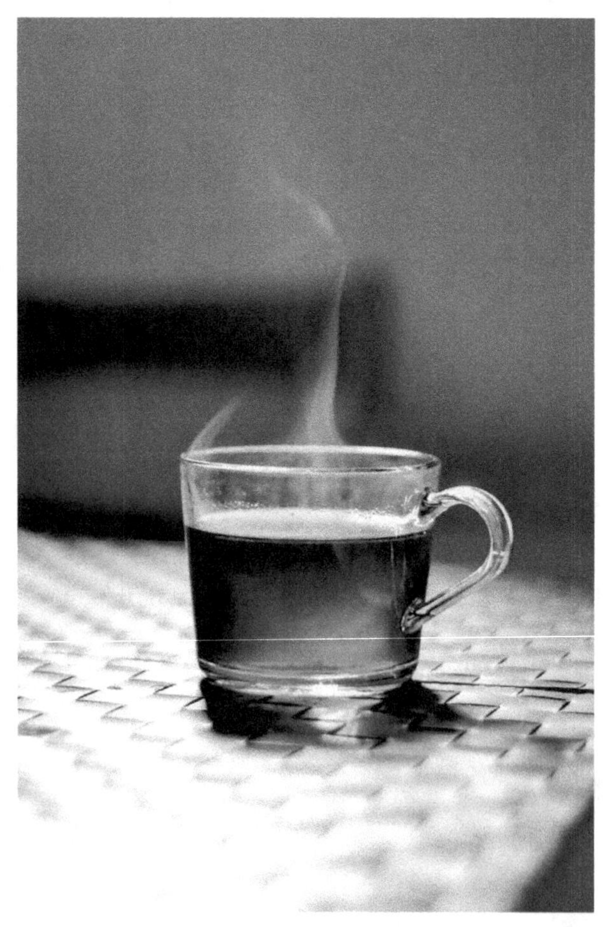

The Pancreas, is essential for your digestion. When the pancreas is overworking hormonal imbalance occurs. Here is how to detox your pancreas naturally.

HOT SHOWER

Taking a hot shower bath improves the health of your pancreas. It will reactivate the functioning of your pancreas.

SCRUB

Scrubbing and bathing with hot water will improve the blood flow to the pancreas. You should scrub your skin gently with a loofah.

EXERCISE

Keep your body moving it will help to eliminate the toxins from your body. This will help with blood circulation of blood to the pancreas.

REDUCE STRESS

Negative emotions, can affect your digestion. Relax, eat healthy and stay hydrated always. Your pancreas will thank you for that.

MEDICINAL PLANTS

Medicinal plants like ginger tea, green tea and licorice tea boosts digestion. They are rich in antioxidants and cleanse your pancreas.

VITAMIN

Take a multivitamin tablet every day. Vitamins help to stimulate the pancreas. It also helps to prevent pancreatic diseases.

CHAPTER EIGHT

DETOX YOUR INTESTINES

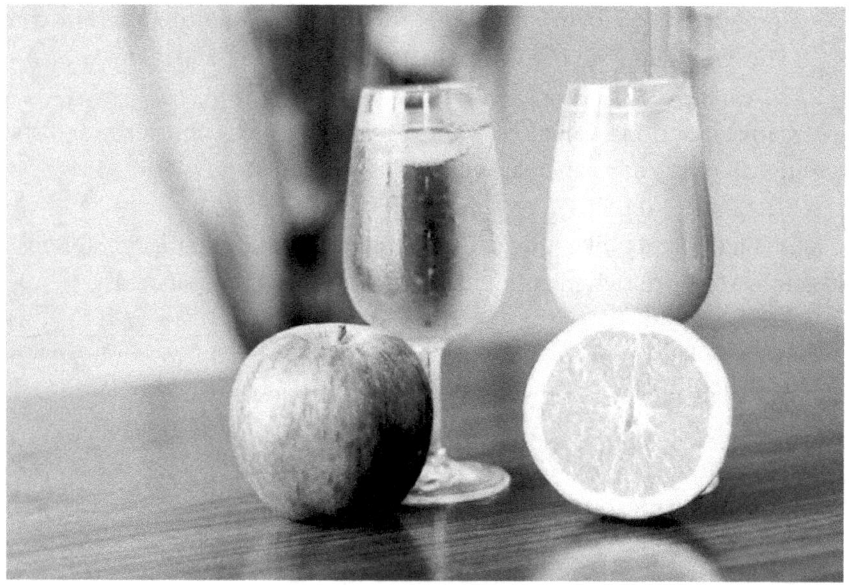

THE LARGE INTESTINE

The large intestine plays a very important role in digestion. A clean large intestine prevents many illnesses.

THE SMALL INTESTINE

The small intestine is the part of our gastrointestinal tract. The absorption of food takes place in our small intestine. The pancreas releases digestive enzymes into the small intestine.

Reduced stomach acid, high antibiotic consumption, organ system dysfunction like liver or kidney disease and diabetes can cause intestinal bacterial overgrowth and may cause mucoid layer.

HOW TO CLEANSE YOUR INTESTINES

EAT MORE FIBRE

Fiber rich food promotes digestion and weight loss. It helps to prevent constipation.

APPLE JUICE

Drinking apple juice, is the best remedy for colon cleansing. It breaks down toxins and improves your liver health. Drink fresh apple juice followed by a glass of water for three days.

PROBIOTIC FOOD

Probiotic rich food can keep your gut healthy. They contain good bacteria which help in absorbing nutrients from your food.

RAW VEGETABLE JUICE

Stay away from cooked food for two days and choose to drink freshly prepared vegetable juice. Green vegetables contain chlorophyll which is beneficial to detox your intestine.

VITAMIN D

Vitamin D can lower your risk of getting cancer. You can get vitamin D by spending ten minutes in the sun. You can also consume vitamin D rich foods like cereals and milk.

DO NOT HOLD BOWEL MOVEMENTS

The build up of fecal matter in your colon, while you hold bowel movement can release toxins and may cause bloating.

ALOE VERA

Aloe Vera, is a natural laxative. It is a great colon cleanser. You can add lemon juice and flax seeds to the juice.

Stay hydrated and exercise regularly. Avoid consuming red meat.

CHAPTER NINE

HOW TO DETOX YOUR BLADDER AND KIDNEYS

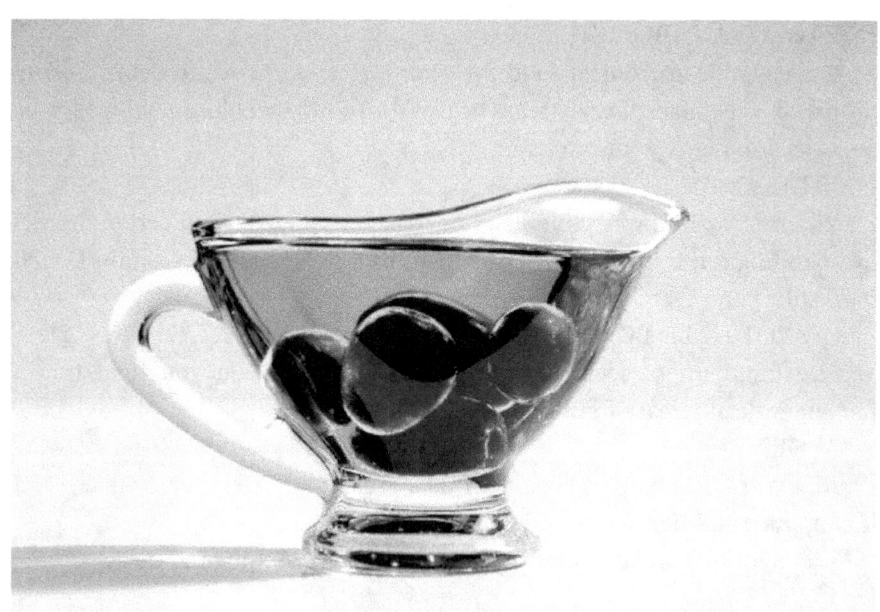

BLADDER

It is important to reduce salt intake to detox your bladder. Bladder, is a very sensitive organ and it plays an important role in storage and elimination of urine.

KIDNEYS

Human has two kidneys. They are bean-shaped organs. They help in fluid balance and hormone secretion. Kidneys filter blood, purify it and remove toxins. Fatigue, swelling in the legs, itching in the body, loss of appetite and dark patches on the skin are signs that your kidneys may have a problem. Here is how to detox your kidneys and bladder.

OLIVE OIL

Olive oil, has anti-inflammatory properties. You can blend a teaspoon of olive oil with a teaspoon of lemon juice and consume. This will help in the prevention of kidney stones.

TURMERIC

Turmeric purifies your blood, liver and kidneys. It has anti-inflammatory properties.

ERADICATE TOXIC FOOD

You should avoid consuming transfat, refined sugars, refined oils and processed food.

POMEGRANATE JUICE

Pomegranate, has astringent properties. This is a best option to detox your kidneys and bladder.

DETOX YOUR KIDNEYS AND BLADDER TWICE A WEEK

You should practice cleansing one day out of three. Don't drink tea, coffee or soda. Avoid sugary beverages. Don't consume protein rich foods. Eat only vegetables, fruits, natural juices and water.

GINGER TEA

Ginger is a spice which detoxifies your bladder and kidneys. It has anti-inflammatory properties and it contains anti-oxidant substances. It also prevents urinary tract infection. You can add it to your food or drink warm ginger tea twice a day.

WATERMELON

Watermelon is great for your bladder. It is a diuretic. It is helpful to prevent urinary system infections.

BARLEY

Barley is full of fiber. It is good for digestion. Soak a handful of barley in water for five hours. Drink this water. It is helpful in weight loss. It acts as a natural cleanser and good for digestion.

TURMERIC, LEMON AND HONEY

Squeeze a slice of lemon into lukewarm water. Add half teaspoon of turmeric in it. Next, add one teaspoon of honey. Stir and consume. This is a perfect blend to get rid of toxins.

BEETROOT

Beetroot is a natural cleanser. It detoxifies the urinary bladder and kidneys of your body.

DRINK COCONUT WATER

Coconut water is the best health drink. It rebalances the electrolytes in your body. It is anti ageing.

You can also drink cucumber juice, carrot juice and Aloe Vera juice with a clove of garlic. Avoid eating chocolate during detoxification.

CHAPTER TEN

NATURAL WAYS TO DETOX YOUR DIGESTIVE SYSTEM

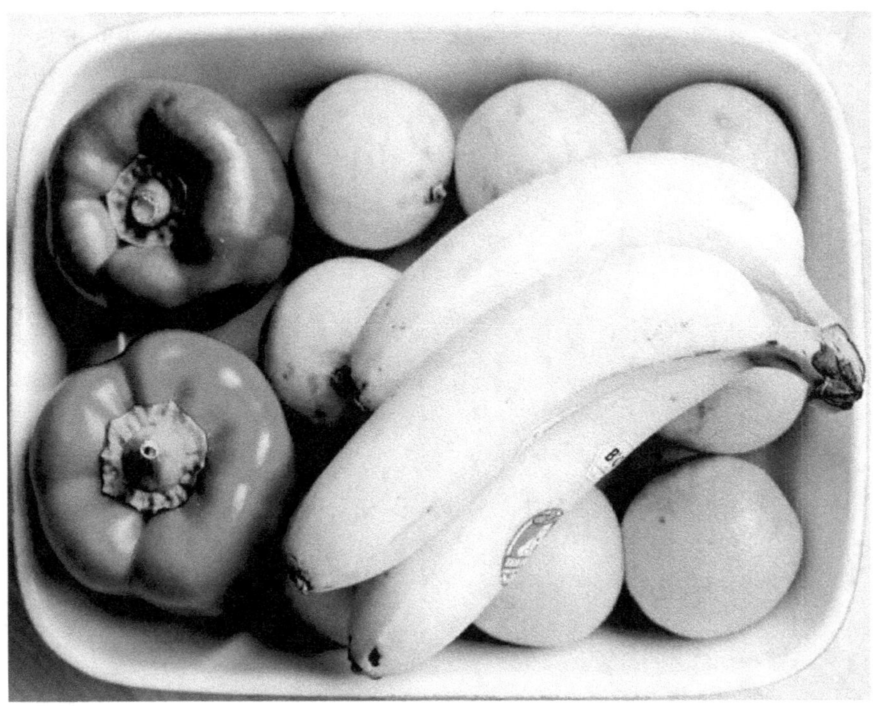

Digestive cleansing is like rebooting your computer. Detoxifying gives your stomach a chance to release all impurities that clog your system. It helps in better absorption of nutrients and help you remain disease free. It also aids in weight loss. When you do a colon cleanse, you will feel light and happy.

FIBROUS FRUIT AND VEGETABLES

The fibre is helpful in cleaning our digestive system. It also helps in slowing down our appetite.

HERBS AND SPICES

Fennel can help reduce bloating and heartburn. Ginger has anti-inflammatory properties. Ginseng boosts your immunity. It will soothe your digestive system. Turmeric will cleanse your liver.

FERMENTED FOODS

Fermented foods are beneficial for our gut health. It eliminates harmful bacteria and improves digestion. Yogurt is a very good option and you can prepare it easily.

WATER

Water eliminates wastes and toxins. It improves digestion, bowel function and increases immunity. It also improves metabolism. Aim to drink eight glasses of water daily.

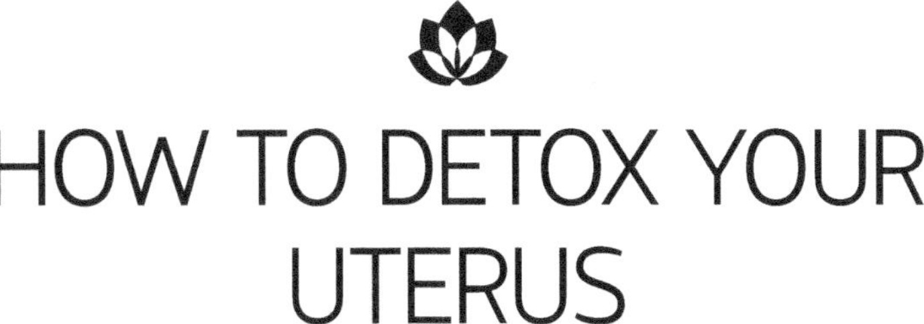

CHAPTER ELEVEN

HOW TO DETOX YOUR UTERUS

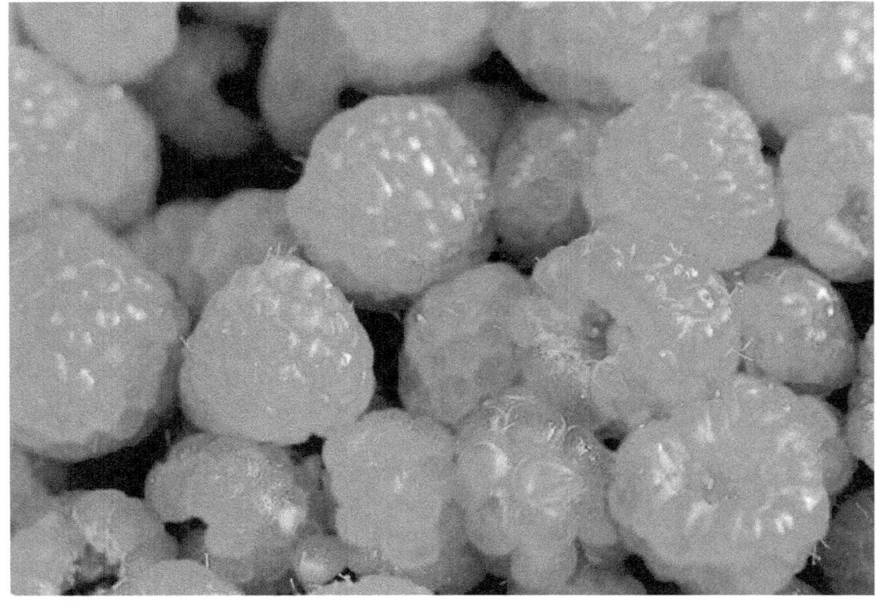

It is important for women, to clean the womb once in a week to avoid fibroids, cysts and many other diseases common in women.

GARLIC

Garlic is the best option to clean your uterus. It has anti-bacterial properties.

FRUITS

Eating a diet rich in fruit may reduce the risk of fibroids, endometriosis and cancer. Fruits contain folic acid.

RED RASPBERRY LEAF

Red raspberry leaf cleans your womb before birth and after birth of your baby. Raspberry leaves are rich in folic acid and nutrients.

BLACKBERRIES

Blackberries are rich in antioxidants. They are also rich in fiber, which helps to get rid of free radicals.

GREEN TEA

Green tea cleans your uterus. It helps in boosting fertility.

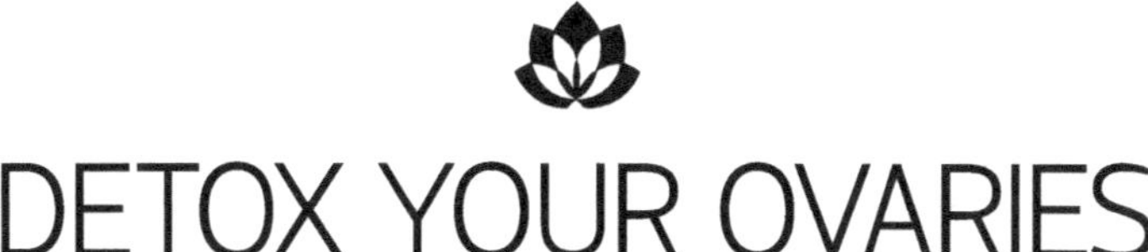

DETOX YOUR OVARIES

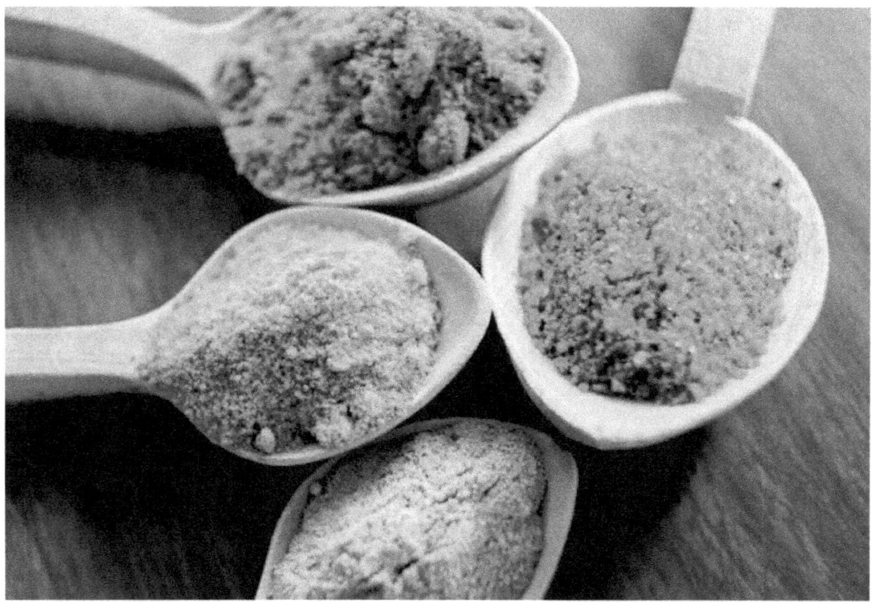

You should clean your ovaries once in a while. This will prevent the cysts. An ovarian cyst is a small fluid filled sac formed in the ovaries. This occurs when the egg is not released or when the sac that the egg was formed in does not dissolve. Here is how to detox your ovaries.

STRENGTHEN YOU LIVER

Your liver is responsible for filtering nutrients and food. It also needs to filter away the toxins and hormones. Go for a liver detox so that your liver filters harmful hormones and lowers the chances of ovarian cysts.

HEAT

Just keep a heating pad on your lower pelvic area and abdomen for half an hour. Do it whenever you feel abdominal pain.

MEDITATION

Get a sufficient amount of quality sleep to handle stress. Turn off all electronics and practice meditation.

EXERCISE

Even a moderate amount of exercise can promote the release of Dopamine, which elevates your mood. This is a solution to prevent ovarian cysts.

CASTOR OILPACK

Castor oil helps in flushing out the excess toxins from your body. It stimulates your lymphatic system and dissolves the ovarian cysts. Don't apply castor oil during your period or ovulation period if you are trying to conceive.

HEALTHY FOOD

Cut back sugar consumption. Drink turmeric milk. Turmeric is rich in minerals and vitamins.

CHAPTER THIRTEEN

DETOX YOUR PENIS

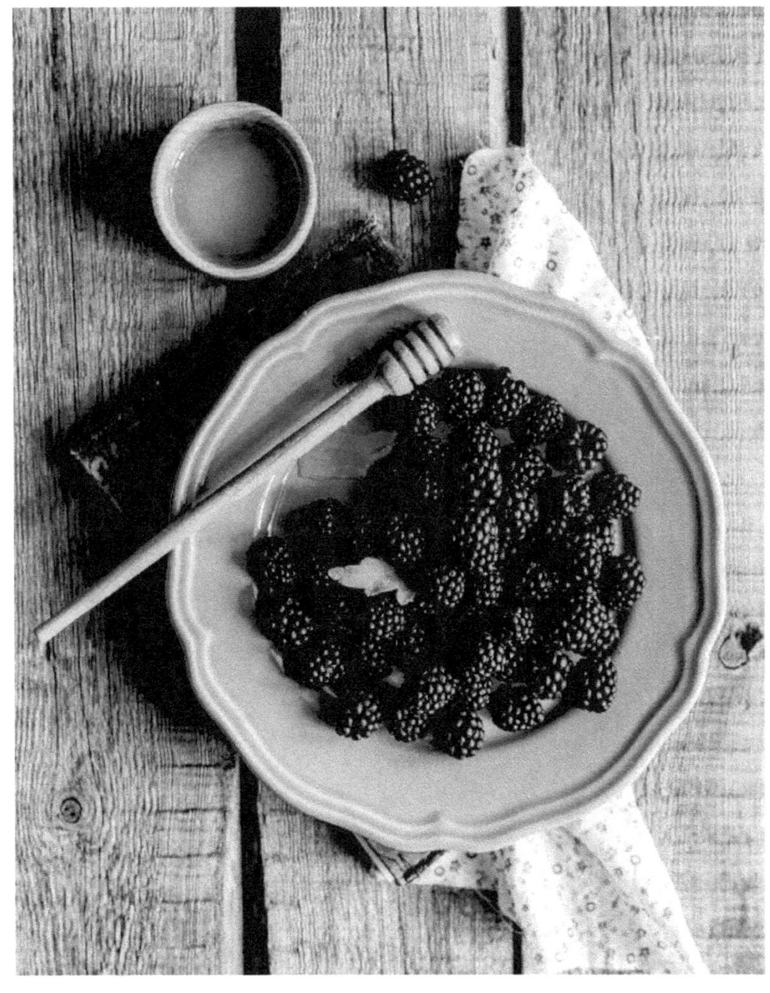

The penis is a sensitive tissue composed of blood vessels. During erection in a man, the blood swifts, to the blood vessels of his penis. You should detox your penis in order to increase blood circulation and boost your stamina. Here is how to detox your penis.

BLACKBERRIES

Blackberries are good for detoxification. They are rich in antioxidants. They are also rich in fibre, which help the body to get rid of toxins.

TURMERIC

Turmeric aids blood circulation, lowers cholesterol and improves blood vessel health. It is used for treatment of obesity.

LICORICE ROOT

Licorice root fights inflammation. It has anti viral and anti bacterial properties. It cleanses the colon.

MILK THISTLE

Milk thistle is good for detoxification. It protects the liver from toxins and pollutants. It prevents free radical damage and stimulates production of new liver cells.

HOW TO DETOX YOUR SKIN

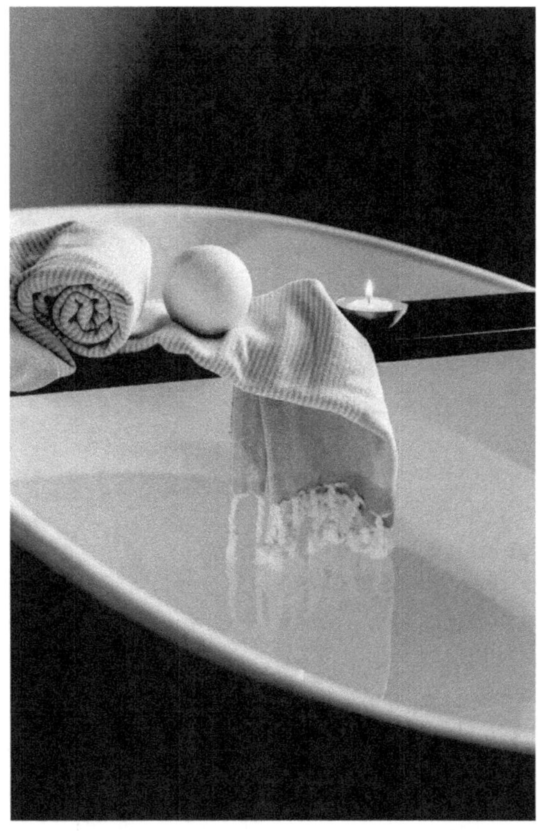

The skin is the body's largest organ. Its main function is protection, regulation and sensation. Your skin will look radiant, when it is detoxified.

Here is how to detox your body at home.

DRY BRUSHING

Brush your skin for five minutes with a dry brush before taking a shower. It helps in removing dead skin cells. It also helps in getting rid of the toxins. Dry brushing stimulates your lymphatic system and aids blood circulation. It helps in reducing the cellulite. Avoid dry brushing your face and your private parts.

DETOX BATH

Here is how to take a detox bath.

GREEN TEA WATER

Take five green tea bags and steep them in your bath water. The water should be hot. Once the water becomes Luke warm take bath in this water or soak yourselves in this water for fifteen minutes if you have got a bathtub.

SEA SALT WATER

Add sea salt to your bathing water. Allow the salt to dissolve in the water. Soak your body for fifteen minutes in this water.

APPLE CIDER VINEGAR

Add one teaspoon of apple cider vinegar and your favourite essential oil to your bathing water. Soak in this water for ten minutes or just take a bath in this water.

COFFEE BATH

Use the coffee powder as a scrub to scrub your body. Allow it to dry. Now, take a warm water bath. You can also mix coffee powder with olive oil.

HOT OIL MASSAGE

Mix equal amount of olive oil and almond oil. You can also add your favourite essential oil. Warm up this mixture and apply all over your body. Leave for half an hour and take a warm water bath. This process helps in detoxifying your skin. It stimulates blood circulation.

Drink plenty of water. Consume fiber and probiotic rich healthy food. Stay away from chemicals and exercise for one hour daily. Sweating aids detoxification. Apply a vitamin C rich cream to tighten and brighten your skin. You can also visit a sauna and take steam for detoxifying your body.

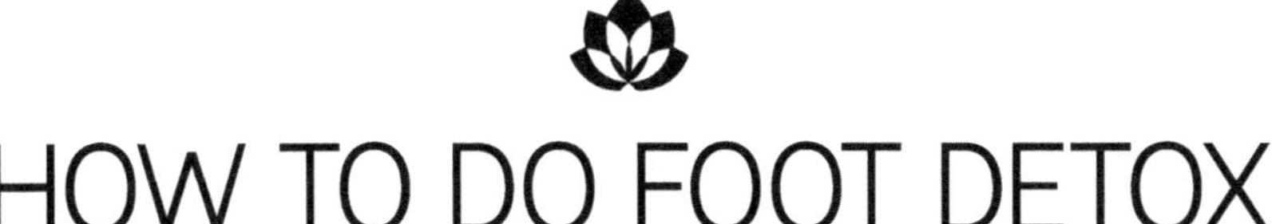

HOW TO DO FOOT DETOX

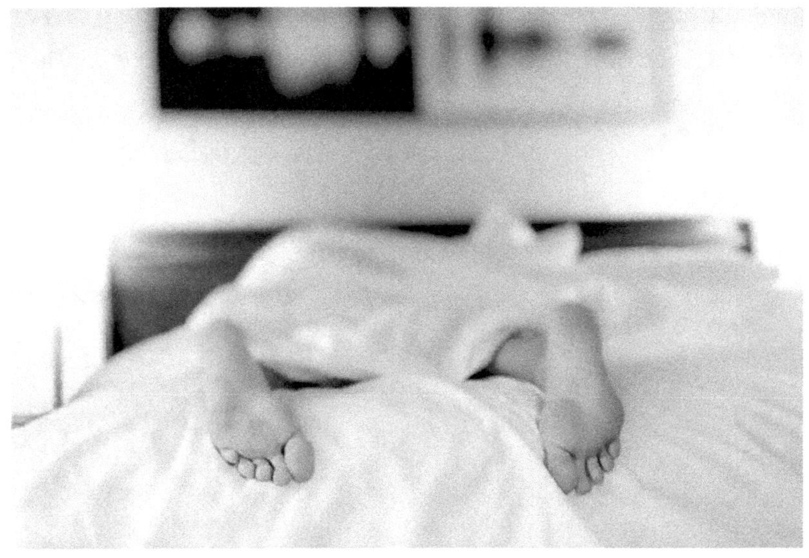

The human body is a composition of innumerable count of cells. It tends to accumulate various impurities and toxins. Detoxification draws out toxic substances and heavy metals from the body and regulates blood circulation. A foot detox can also aid detoxification and remove toxins from your blood through your feet. It can eliminate heavy metals, balance the pH levels, relieve stress, uplift mood, reduce inflammation, aid weight loss and keep your heart healthy. Here is how to do a foot detox.

FOOT SOAK

Add two tablespoons salt to half bucket of warm water. Add a few drops of your favourite essential oils. Soak your feet in this water for some time. You can also use apple cider vinegar, Epsom salt or baking soda instead of salt.

FOOT MASK

Apply a clay foot mask. It cleanses and exfoliates your feet. Wash after some time.

FOOT SCRUB

Foot scrubs soften your feet. It removes foot odour and dead skin cells. It helps in easing pain. You can also take a foot massage after scrubbing.

FOOT PADS

Foot pads are useful in pulling out toxins. It aids sweating.

ACCUPRESSURE

Pressing specific points of your feet helps in reducing tension. It promotes relaxation.

CHAPTER SIXTEEN

HOW TO MAKE HOMEMADE DETOX FOOT PADS

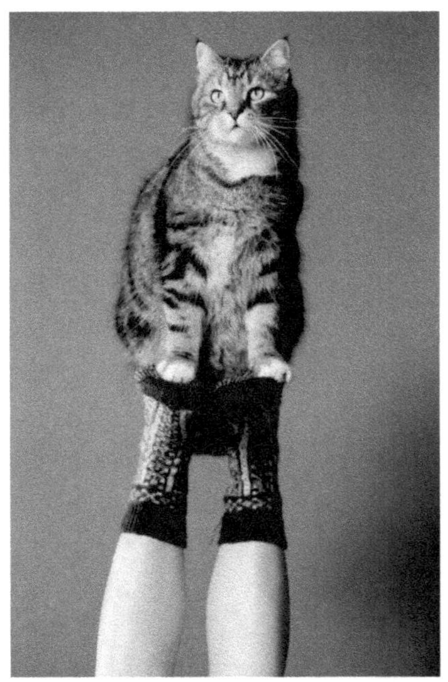

Foot pads stimulate the liver and kidney. It increases her metabolic rate of your liver and kidney. It detoxifies your blood and body. Here is how to prepare foot detox pads at home.

INGREDIENTS

Garlic paste – One teaspoon

Onion paste – One teaspoon

Apple cider vinegar – Half cup

Socks

Gauze pads

Saucepan

METHOD OF PREPARATION AND APPLICATION

Bring Apple cider vinegar to boil. Add onion and garlic paste. Allow it to steep for ten minutes. Remove the solution from the heat. Allow it to cool. Pour the solution on gauze pads. Squeeze out the excess fluid. Apply the gauze pads on your feet. Put on your socks and go to sleep. Peel the pad in the morning, next pad.

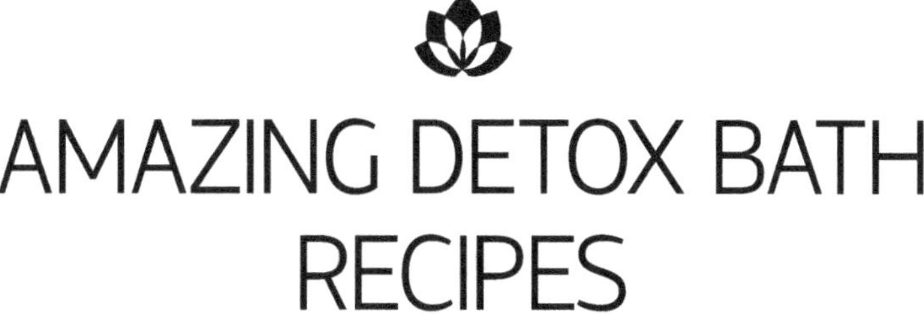

CHAPTER SEVENTEEN

AMAZING DETOX BATH RECIPES

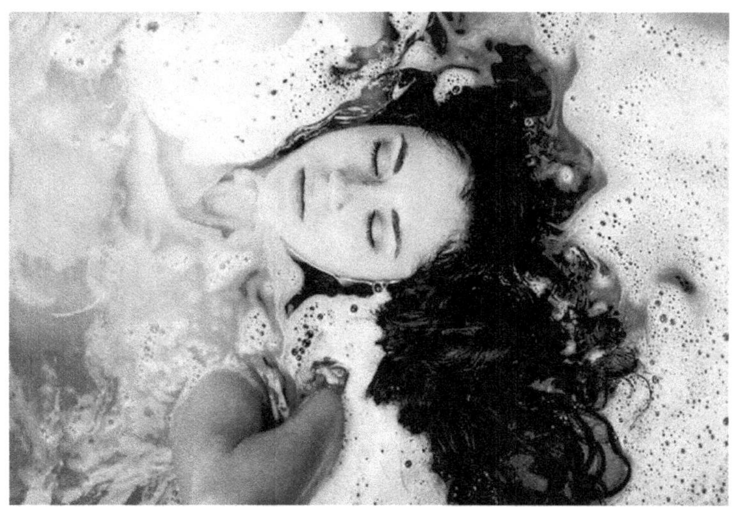

Nothing is more is relaxing than trying these detox bath recipes. These detox bath recipes help in removing excess toxins from the body. It is an inexpensive way to boost your health. Here is how to prepare the amazing detox bath recipes.

OXYGEN DETOX BATH RECIPES

INGREDIENTS TO BE TAKEN

Hydrogen peroxide – two cups

Ginger – one piece grated or ground

METHOD OF PREPARATION

Fill the tub with warm water. Add the hydrogen peroxide and ginger paste. Soak in the tub for half an hour.

HOMEMADE MILK BATH

INGREDIENTS NEEDED

Coconut milk – One cup

Your favourite essential oil – A few drops

METHOD OF BATHING

Add one cup of coconut milk and a few drops of your favourite essential oil to your bathing water. Soak yourself in this water for half an hour. You can also use almond milk instead of coconut milk. You can also massage this mixture on your body and leave for half an hour before taking bath.

You can take a detox bath once in a week, but not more than that. Ensure that you drink plenty of water while taking a detox bath.

CHAPTER EIGHTEEN

DETOX SHAMPOO RECIPES FOR HAIR

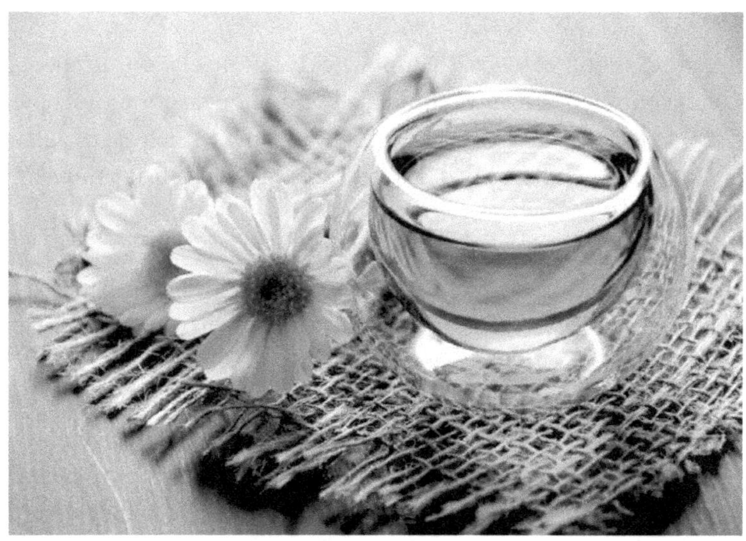

Our tresses are exposed to pollution. Here are great detox shampoo recipes for your hair.

LEMON AND CUCUMBER

Peel one cucumber. Blend it in a blender to make a smooth paste. Add one teaspoon lemon juice to this paste. Apply on your hair and massage well. Wash and rinse thoroughly. Lemon is a cleaner and cucumber is a cooler.

COFFFEE AND SALT SHAMPOO

Mix one teaspoon of coffee grounds with one teaspoon of sea salt and one teaspoon of baby shampoo. Mix all the ingredients and make a paste. Apply this on your scalp and massage for ten minutes. Rinse with plain water. Do this twice a week.

BAKING SODA

Put one tablespoon of baking soda in a mug of water. You can also add your favourite essential oils and a teaspoon of sea salt to this water. Massage well into your scalp. You can wash your hair with baby shampoo. Rinse your scalp and hair with vinegar and finally with water. It will make your hair silky.

HONEY SHAMPOO

Add a few drops of Lavender essential oil to two tablespoons of honey. Massage it on your wet hair. This shampoo will clean your hair and control your frizzy hair as well.

COCONUT OIL AND SALT SHAMPOO

Mix one teaspoon of baby shampoo with one teaspoon of coconut oil. Add one teaspoon of Himalayan pink salt and one teaspoon of Apple cider vinegar. Mix all the ingredients and apply to your wet hair. Massage for ten minutes. Rinse with normal water. Coconut oil is rich in vitamins and it is ideal for dry hair.

COCONUT MILK AND ALOE VERA

Apply a paste of coconut milk and Aloe Vera on your wet hair. Aloe Vera helps to get rid of dandruff. Use this like your normal shampoo. Coconut milk contains proteins and it restores the natural oil.

FULLER"S EARTH AND SEA SALT SHAMPOO

Mix two teaspoons of fuller's earth with one teapsoon of sea salt. Add this to one teaspoon of baby shampoo and one teaspoon of olive oil. Mix and make a paste. Apply this on your scalp. Massage your hair for five minutes. Rinse with plain water. This wil give your hair a bouncy look. The fuller's earth absorbs all the dirt and cleans your scalp.

CINNAMON MASK

Mix one teaspoon of cinnamon with one teaspoon of baking soda and two teaspoons of olive oil. Massage this mixture to your hair and scalp. Leave it in for half an hour. Rinse your hair. This mask pulls out grime and build-up. It is high in antioxidants.

CHAPTER NINETEEN

INDIAN DETOX MEAL PLANS

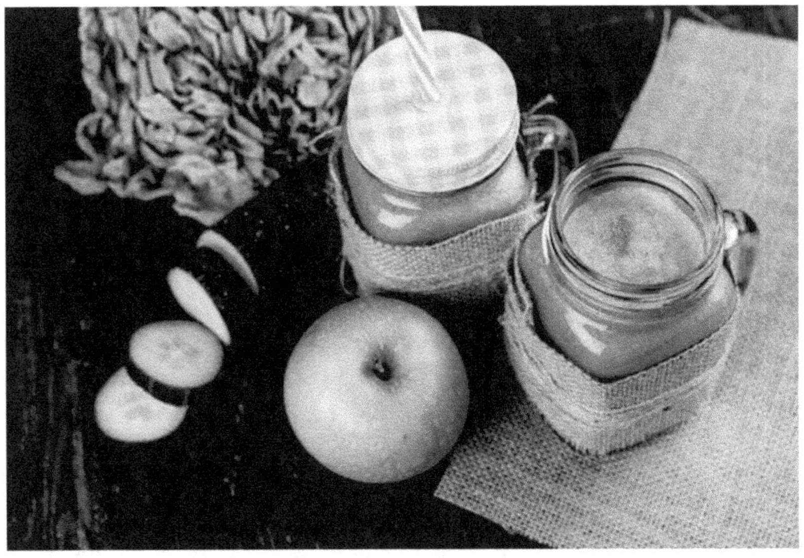

A cleanse program is a tool to rejuvenate your body. You will have to eliminate sugar, alcohol, fats and processed foods while detoxification and consume fibre rich fruits, vegetables and plenty of water. Here is a detox diet plan.

DAY 1

Start your day by drinking warm lemon water.

BREAKFAST

One glass of fresh vegetable juice. (Carrot, beetroot, coriander, one teaspoon of Chia seed and wheatgrass)

LUNCH

Steamed vegetables. (Mushroom, Beetroot, Pumpkins, Onion, garlic and ginger)

SNACKS

Drink as much as herbal tea. Mixture of nuts and roasted seeds.

DINNER

Vegetable stew

Saute onions and garlic. Add your favourite vegetables.

DAY 2

Start your day with warm lemon water.

BREAKFAST

Fresh vegetable juice with one teaspoon of Chia seed sprinkled over it.

LUNCH

Lightly cooked vegetables with half cup Quinoa.

SNACKS

Nuts and roasted seeds.

DINNER

Vegetable stew with yellow and red capsicum, extra virgin olive oil, lemon juice and garlic.

DAY 3

Start the morning with a glass of freshly squeezed lemon juice added to warm water.

BREAKFAST

Natural yogurt with fruits and Chia seeds sprinkled over it. You can also add almonds, raw honey and walnuts. You can also have green tea.

LUNCH

Lentil and vegetable stew. (Saute half cup moong dal, one cup of vegetables, small pieces of garlic and ginger with extra virgin olive oil.)

SNACKS

Nuts and roasted seeds.

DINNER

Raw papapya and carrot salad. You can also add one teaspoon of lemon juice and extra virgin olive oil to the salad.

DAY 4

Start the morning with warm lemon water. You can also do yoga, brisk walking or swimming.

BREAKFAST

Coconut banana smoothie.

Take 100 grams of coconut milk and one cup of sliced banana. Mix them and add a teaspoon of Chia seeds to it.

LUNCH

One bowl of vegetables.

SNACKS

One handful nuts and seeds mixture.

DINNER

Lentil and vegetable stew.

DAY 5

Start your day by drinking warm lemon water. You can do yoga, brisk walking or swimming.

BREAKFAST

Fresh vegetable juice with one teaspoon of Sunflower seeds added.

LUNCH

Steamed vegetables seasoned with olive oil. You can have this curry with brown rice.

SNACKS

A handful of nuts.

DINNER

Salad of red and yellow capsicum, mushrooms and onion. Sprinkle one teaspoon Flax seeds. Season with Olive oil.

DAY 6

Start the morning with a glass of warm lemon water. Do brisk walking, yoga or swimming.

BREAKFAST

You can have apple pieces added to yogurt and a teaspoon of flaxseeds sprinkled on it.

LUNCH

Lentil with vegetable soup. Brown rice with vegetable stir fry.

SNACKS

Nuts and roasted seeds.

DINNER

Raw papaya and carrot sticks.

DAY 7

Start the morning with warm lemon water. Do yoga, brisk walking or swimming.

BREAKFAST
Coconut banana smoothie.
LUNCH
Lentil and vegetable soup.
SNACKS
Nuts and roasted seeds.
DINNER
Mushroom and sweet potato stir fry with half cup brown rice.

Congrats, you have finished your seven days cleanse. You will be feeling fantastic. Your skin will be glowing and you will be looking fresh and rejuvenated.

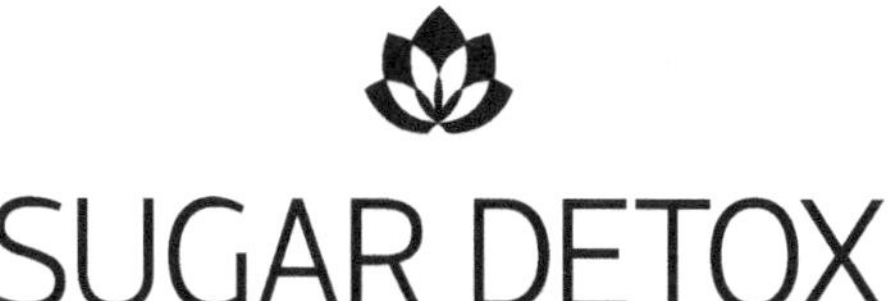

CHAPTER TWENTY

SUGAR DETOX

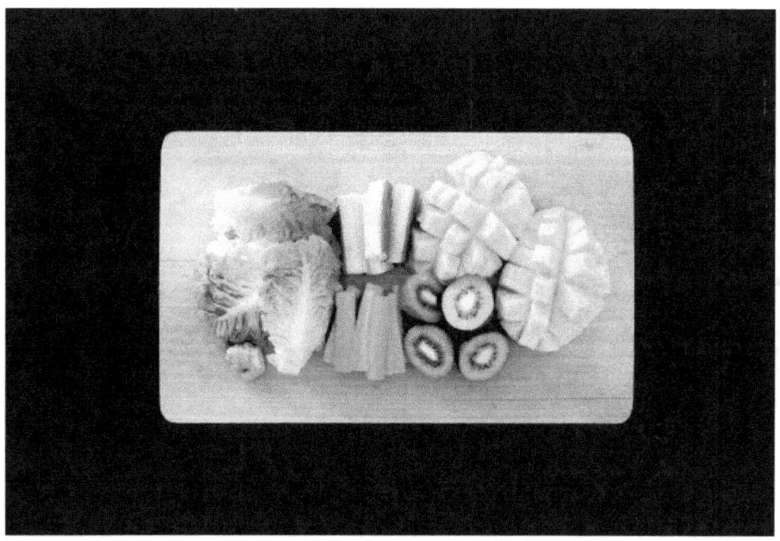

Fat doesn't make you fat. Sugar makes you fat. You need a sugar detox because sugar is an addictive substance. A sugar detox will break the addiction. Once you eliminate sugar from your diet, your body will adapt to the lack. Breaking an addiction, may cause withdrawal symptoms like headache or cravings. Before you feel better it may make you feel worse. You may also notice a low mood, anxiety, nausea, fatigue and concentration problems. All the side effects are temporary and the benefits of sugar detox of our body is really worth the sacrifice. You need to quit sugar for three weeks, during a sugar detox period. Here is how to follow a sugar detox diet.

DIET

Avoid sugary drinks, soda and artificial sweeteners. Drink hydrating beverages like water, detox water or vegetable juice. Fruit has natural sugars. Replace desserts with fruits. Fruits are rich in antioxidants. Healthy fat sources help in reducing cravings. Increase the consumption of healthy fats like nuts and seeds. Increase protein consumption. Eat a protein rich food in your breakfast. Don't forget to consume veggies. Olives are good for detoxification. You can consume them as snacks. Don't skip your meals. Avoid potato, sweet potato and beets while doing sugar detox.

GLUTAMINE SUPPLEMENT

Glutamine is an amino acid. We can consume it in supplement form. It helps to control cravings and regulates our blood sugar levels.

SLEEP

You may feel tired while on a sugar detox. You should good quality sleep of eight hours.

CAN I EAT SUGAR AFTER DETOX?

Yes, but it is better to switch to natural sugars.

CHAPTER TWENTY-ONE

WEEKEND DETOX

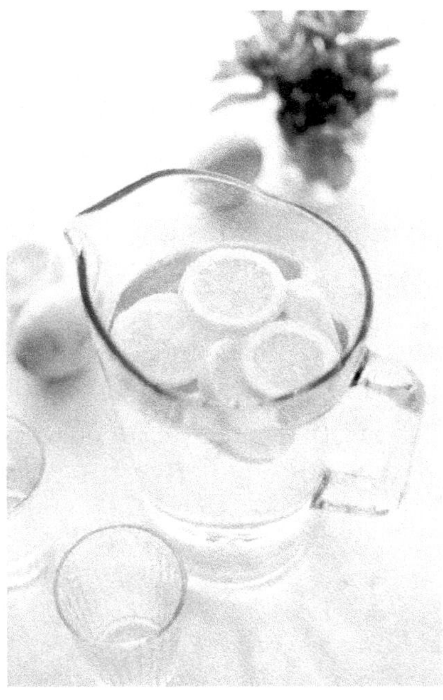

You may need a good night's sleep on Friday night if you have planned for a weekend detox. Here is how to do a weekend detox.

DAY ONE

YOGA

Wake up and do yoga for half an hour. You can do some stretching and bending asanas.

LEMON WATER

Prepare a pitcher of lemon water. Drink a glass of warm lemon water early in the morning. It stimulates the bowels and helps in detoxifying your liver. Keep sipping a glass of lemon water every one hour throughout the day. Do not consume tea or coffee. You can have green tea or Dandelion tea as it aids detoxification.

DRY BRUSH YOUR BODY

Dry brush stimulates the lymphatic system. Start from your toes towards your heart. Follow with a warm water shower. It boosts blood circulation.

BREAKFAST

You can have steamed vegetables like carrot and sweet potato. You can listen to a music, meditate or read a book after your breakfast to relieve your stress.

LUNCH

You can have a vegetable salad in the lunch. After lunch you have to go for a short brisk walk to keep your blood circulating well. Sweating helps in eliminating the toxins. You can also take a massage and steam bath.

TAKE A NAP

You can take a short nap after taking steam bath. You can again consume a bowl of vegetables in the snack time.

DINNER

You can have a lentil and vegetable salad with a dash of pepper. After dinner you can again listen to music, read a book or do whatever interests you. You can drink a calming Chamomile tea or one teaspoon Psyllium seed dissolved in half cup of water. It helps in bowel movement.

Repeat the same routine on day two.

CHAPTER TWENTY-TWO

DETOX SMOOTHIE RECIPES

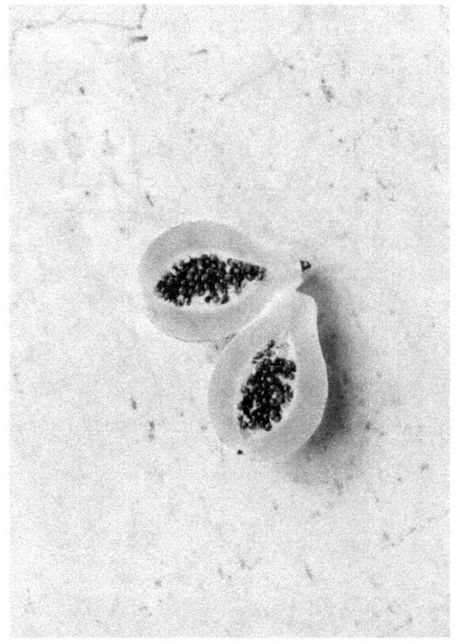

Detox Smoothies flush out toxins from your body and have tremendous health benefits. You can have them in between meals. Here is how to prepare a detox smoothie.

PAPAYA LIVER CLEANSE SMOOTHIE

Cut a papaya to pieces. Blend it in a blender along with seeds. Enjoy this liver cleanse drink.

COCOA SMOOTHIE

Mix one teaspoon of Cocoa powder with half cup of coconut milk and half cup of strawberries. Blend all the ingredients in a blender. Pour this drink in a glass and enjoy.

MANGO BANANA PAPAYA SMOOTHIE

Take one small katori of mango chunks, banana slices and papaya pieces. Blend it in a blender and drink this healthy drink.

STRAWBERRY AND BEETROOT DETOX SMOOTHIE

Beetroots purify your body. They are rich in fiber. They encourage cell regeneration. Chia seeds are packed with nutrition and they aid digestion. You have to grate one cup of beet-root. Blend it in a blender with half cup of strawberry pieces and one teaspoon of Chia seed. Enjoy this smoothie.

PINEAPPLE SMOOTHIE

Take a few pieces of Pineapple and mix with half cup coconut milk and a teaspoon of Cinnamon. Blend in a blender. Enjoy this drink.

APPLE SMOOTHIE RECIPE

Blend a few pieces of apples, half cup coconut milk and a teaspoon of cinnamon powder in a blender. Enjoy the drink.

MANGO SMOOTHIE RECIPE

Blend a few pieces of mango with half cup yogurt. Enjoy this healthy drink.

STRAWBERRY SMOOTHIE RECIPE

Mix one bowl of banana slices with one bowl of chopped strawberries. Enjoy this quick and healthy drink.

KITCHARI CLEANSING DIET

Kitchari cleansing diet can improve your digestion, remove toxins from your system, encourage a balanced sleep cycle and promote overall health. During the three-day cleanse diet, you will be eating only kitchari and oatmeal. You can garnish your kitchari with coriander leaves and sesame seeds. Try to eat before 7 p.m. Drink ten to twelve glasses of water in a day. Don't follow this diet during your periods. This diet is beneficial during Panchkarma treatment. This diet helps to rejuvenate your body and balance the three doshas of our body.

DAILY ROUTINE TO FOLLOW DURING THE THREE DAY CLEANSE

Wake up early in the morning. Scrape your tongue and brush your teeth. Drink four glasses of warm water. Stretch your body and exercise or do yoga. Take a self oil massage and warm bath shower. You can also take a detox bath. Eat Kitchari in the breakfast and lunch. You can take liquids between the meals. You can drink herbal tea as much as you want, but you should quit caffeine consumption. Take one teaspoon of Triphala juice in warm water. Have Kitchari at 7 p.m. Get eight hours of undisturbed sleep. Follow this for three days.

KITCHARI RECIPE

INGREDIENTS

Basmati rice – one cup

Yellow mung dal – half cup

Cardamom – 4 pods

Cinnamon – one stick

Ghee – two tablespoons

Turmeric powder and cumin seeds – half teaspoon

Coriander powder – one teaspoon

Ginger paste – one teaspoon

Asafoetida – one pinch

Two cups of vegetables – carrot and beans.

Shredded coconut – half cup

Coriander leaves.

Salt and pepper according to taste.

METHOD OF PREPARATION

Soak mung dal for four hours. Warm the ghee and add the spices and ginger. Add the soaked mung dal, vegetables, coconut and rice. Add six glasses of water and salt. Stir well. Cover and cook thoroughly, garnish and enjoy with coriander chutney or sesame chutney. You can sprinkle pepper according to your taste.

Blend one bunch of coriander leaves with half cup coconut and a small piece of ginger to prepare coriander chutney. Add a teaspoon of lemon juice.

CHAPTER TWENTY-FOUR

SUPERFOODS FOR DETOXIFICATION

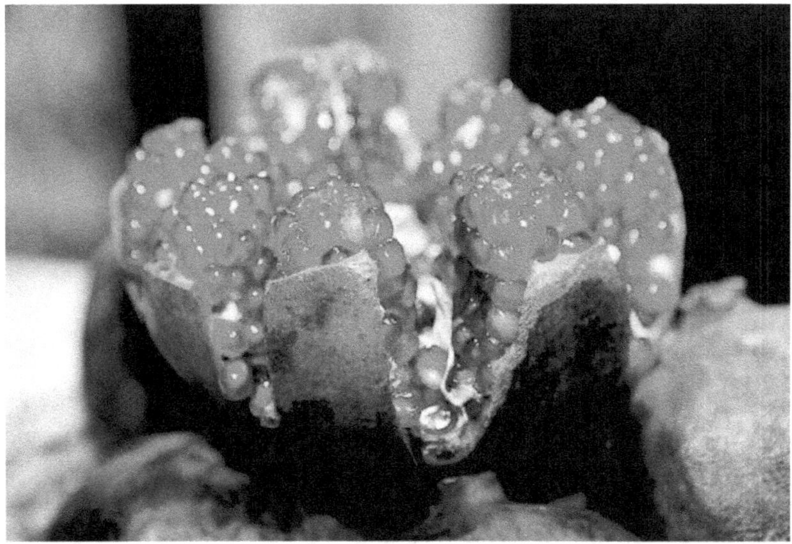

Detoxification is removing toxins from our body and blood. There are many super foods which help in detoxification. Here are some super foods for detoxification.

MILK THISTLE

Milk thistle is good for detoxification. It is packed with flavanoid silymarin which rejuvenates your liver. Milk thistle promotes healthy digestion and reduces inflammation. It is recommended if you have liver cirrhosis, fatty liver, chronic hepatitis and toxicity. Milk thistle elevates good cholesterol and lowers blood pressure. It also regenerates the cells of your kidneys. It protects against radiation damage, cancer, UV radiation damage, diabetes and environment toxins. Milk thistle slows down ageing and reduces cell damage. You can consume milk thistle supplements by taking your doctor's advice.

ALOE VERA

Aloe Vera has anti inflammatory, anti bacterial and soothing properties. It is packed with antioxidants and vitamins. Aloe Vera can cleanse your kidneys, liver, large intestine and can fight cancer. It cleanses your body naturally and supports weight loss. It lowers your cholesterol and improves your digestion. Aloe Vera is also helpful in strengthening your immune system. Here is how to prepare Aloe Vera juice.

Add two tablespoons of Aloe Vera pulp to a glass of water. Add one teaspoon of lemon juice. Drink this twice a day. You can also add it orange juice or coconut water.

POMEGRANATE

Pomegranate is rich in vitamins and antioxidants. It reduces dangerous cholesterol. It lowers blood pressure. Pomegranate aids weight loss, helps to combat water retention, helps in liver detox, helps with diabetes, relieves constipation, treats cancer, boosts memory and sexual performance. It is good for your skin and has anti-microbial properties. It also helps hair growth.

PINEAPPLE

Pineapple has diuretic properties. It is a rich source of antioxidants. It reduces the risk of cardiovascular diseases, improves bone health, promotes digestion, aids weight loss and supports your immune system.

CARROT

Carrots are alkaline in nature. They can reverse acidity. It can protect you from cancer, improve your skin health, well for your eyes and it cleanses your system.

SPIRULINA

Spirulina will replenish your blood cells, boost your energy, eliminate bad breath and act as a natural deodorant. It protects your liver. You can consume a Spirulina supplement after consulting your doctor.

WHEAT GRASS

Wheat grass is packed with Chlorophyll. It cleanses your blood. It helps with digestion. It is beneficial for people with diabetes, obesity and stress.

It improves your skin tone.

LEMON GRASS

Lemon grass is a diuretic. It relieves insomnia, eliminates body odour, aids weight loss, cure diabetes, regulates your blood pressure, promotes digestion and cures yeast infection. It is good for your dental health as it has anti-microbial properties. It balances the PH of your blood.

COCONUT WATER

Coconut water repairs all the tissues of your body. It is helpful in eliminating all the toxins from your body and brightens your skin tone. It purifies the blood and improves digestion. Coconut water lowers your blood pressure and cholesterol. It also relieves muscle stress and is good for athletes.

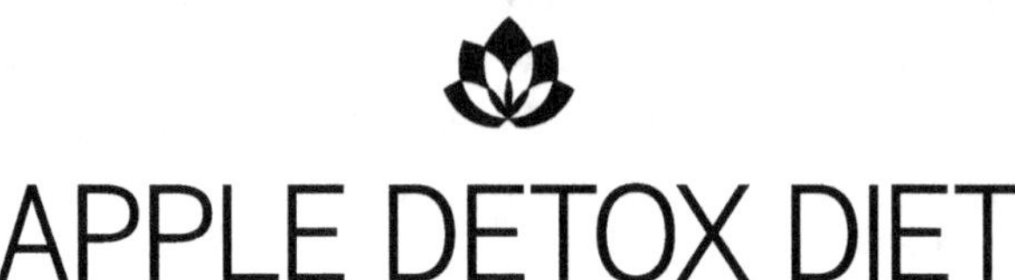

CHAPTER TWENTY-FIVE

APPLE DETOX DIET

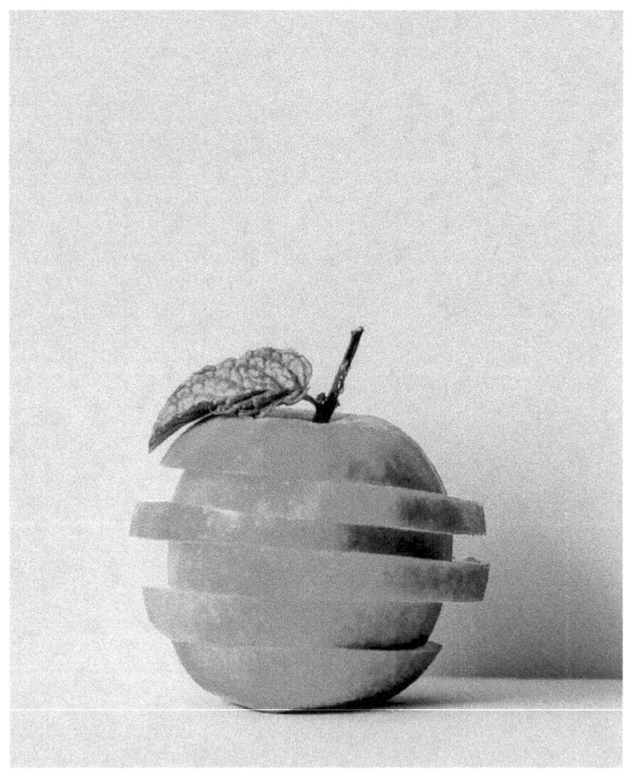

Apples contain fibre. Eating an apple is a healthy option. They are rich in nutrients and antioxidants. Apple is great for your skin. It reduces your cholesterol level. The apple detox diet alkalizes your body and purifies your blood. Here is how to do the apple detox diet.

DAYS 1, 2 AND 3

You will consume only green juice, steamed vegetables and fruits. You can have a half cup of quinoa. You should not eat after 7 PM.

DAYS 3, 4 AND 5

You can eat as much apples as you want and drink as much herbal tea as you want. You can do meditation and take detox baths.

DAYS 6 AND 7

You can consume green juice, steamed vegetables and fruits. You can have a small meal. You can have protein rich curry seasoned with olive oil.

You may feel sleepy during the detox period. You may also feel weak. Drink enough water and stay hydrated. You should drink two litres of water per day during this detox. You can lose about five kilos by this diet. Ensure that you get enough sleep while following this diet plan. You may experience headache and irritability. This diet is not for pregnant or lactating women.

CHAPTER TWENTY-SIX

THE PINEAPPLE DETOX DIET

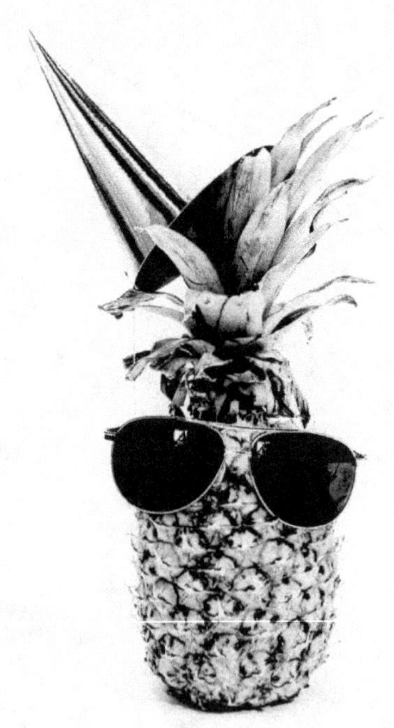

You can lose weight and detox with the pineapple detox diet. Pineapple is rich in fibre. It is a diuretic and improves digestion. Pineapple contains

Bromelain, which helps to absorb nutrients. It improves our eye sight. Pineapple reduces cardiovascular diseases, relieves symptoms of arthritis and improves bone health. Use fresh pineapple for pineapple detox diet. Here is how to do.

BREAKFAST

Pineapple with yogurt and a few almonds

SNACK

One glass of pineapple juice

LUNCH

Steamed vegetables of your choice (Tomato, mushroom etc.)

SNACK

One glass of pineapple juice

DINNER

Pineapple salad and sprout salad with one bowl of yogurt

Stick to this menu for five days. Don't follow this diet plan if you have any health issues. You will lose five to seven kilos by this diet. You should use a ripe pineapple for this diet plan. Don't add sugar to pineapple juice. You can add lemon juice and pepper to pineapple juice. You can drink as much as pineapple water you want. Here is how to prepare detox pineapple water.

PINEAPPLE WATER

INGREDIENTS NEEDED

Pineapple

Water

Honey

Cinnamon

One piece of ginger, grated.

METHOD OF PREPARATION

Boil one liter of water. Add peeled pineapple skin. Add one teaspoon cinnamon and the grated ginger. Boil it for thirty minutes. Add honey. Freeze for one hour. Serve.

Pineapple water aids weight loss and helps to get rid of body fat.

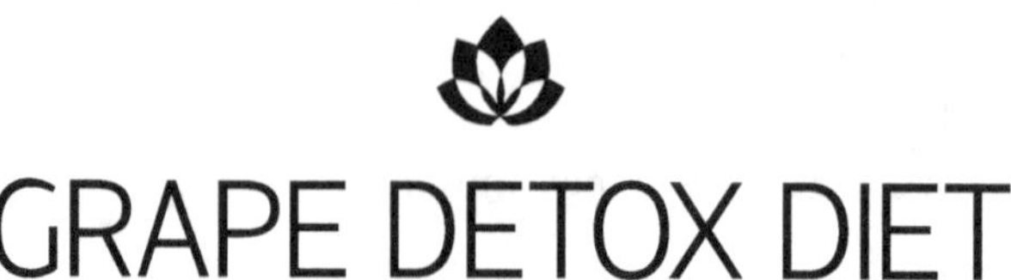

CHAPTER TWENTY-SEVEN

GRAPE DETOX DIET

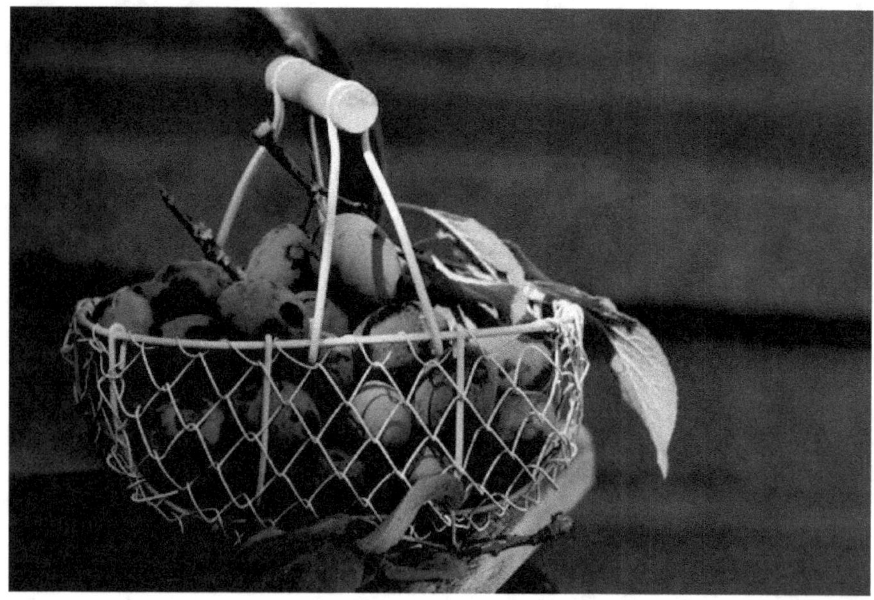

Grapes are rich in antioxidants. They are packed with vitamins and minerals. Grapes are rich in Resveratrol an antioxidant which is beneficial in preventing strokes, heart disease and cancer. Grape detox diet should be followed for four days. You many experience temporary side effect like headache during this detox period. Here is how to do a grape detox diet.

DAY ONE

BREAKFAST

Grapes added to one bowl of yogurt

LUNCH
Grape and vegetable salad
DINNER
Fruit salad with lots of grapes
DAY TWO
BREAKFAST
One glass of grape juice
SNACK
One bowl of yogurt
LUNCH
One bowl of grapes and vegetable salad
DINNER
Fruit salad with lots of grapes
DAY THREE
BREAKFAST
One bowl of grapes with one cheese sandwich
LUNCH
One bowl of steamed vegetable and one bowl of grapes
DINNER
One bowl of fruit salad with lots of grapes
DAY FOUR
BREAKFAST
One bowl of grapes with one cheese sandwich
LUNCH
One bowl of grapes
DINNER
One bowl of steamed vegetables and grape salad (Carrot, mushroom and grapes)

CHAPTER TWENTY-EIGHT

ARMPIT DETOX AND BREAST DETOX FOODS

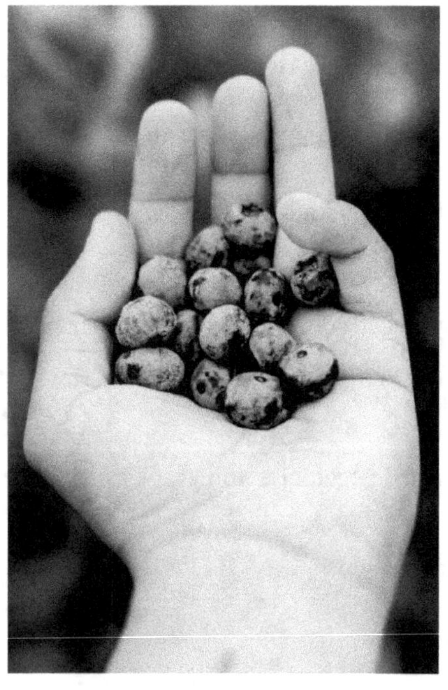

Breast cancer happens due to genetics, environmental toxins or due to wrong lifestyle. Here is how to detoxify your breasts. Some foods are helpful for your breast health. Here are some super foods for your breast health.
VITAMIN D

Vitamin D is essential to strengthen our immunity. You can get it from sunlight.

OLIVE OIL

Extra virgin olive oil is rich in antioxidants. It prevents breast cancer.

OMEGA 3 FATTY ACIDS

Walnuts, pumpkin seeds, flax seeds, etc are rich in Omega 3 fatty acids. You should eat turnips, cruciferous vegetables and green leafy vegetables.

TURMERIC

Turmeric arrests the spread of breast cancer. It reduces the damaging effect of chemotherapy.

BLUEBERRY

Blueberries decrease tumour growth. They can be added to yogurt or smoothies.

GREEN TEA

It is rich in antioxidants. It strengthens your immunity.

IODINE

Iodine is required for both thyroid and breast. It is known to kill cancer cells.

PLANT BASED PROTEIN

Legumes and lentils are rich in protein. They are also rich in antioxidants and very effective in preventing cancer.

THINGS GOOD FOR YOUR BREAST HEALTH

Massage

Sipping hot water

Dry brushing of the body

Detox baths

Fibre rich diet

Quit smoking and consuming alcohol. Reduce your weight and exercise. Breast feeding prevents breast cancer. Avoid exposure to environmental chemicals.

HOW TO DETOX YOUR ARMPIT

Aluminium causes breast cancer. You should avoid deodorants and stick to natural option to detox your armpits. Here is how to detox your armpits.

SCRUB

Scrub your underarms with a loofah. You can do this while having a shower.

BAKING SODA

Apply Baking soda to your armpits while they are still wet. Wash once and apply again.

LEMON JUICE

Instead of Baking soda, you can also clean your armpits with lemon juice. It cleans your armpits and kills the bacteria. It improves the body odour.

Avoid razors and hot wax as it may irritate your skin.